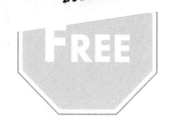

D1600393

FREE
DVD

FREE
DVD

From Stress to Success DVD
from Trivium Test Prep

Dear Customer,

Thank you for purchasing from Trivium Test Prep! Whether you're looking to join the military, get into college, or advance your career, we're honored to be a part of your journey.

To show our appreciation (and to help you relieve a little of that test-prep stress), we're offering a **FREE *MBLEx Essential Test Tips DVD*** by Trivium Test Prep. Our DVD includes 35 test preparation strategies that will help keep you calm and collected before and during your big exam. All we ask is that you email us your feedback and describe your experience with our product. Amazing, awful, or just so-so: we want to hear what you have to say!

To receive your **FREE *MBLEx Test Tips DVD***, please email us at 5star@ triviumtestprep.com. Include "Free 5 Star" in the subject line and the following information in your email:

1. The title of the product you purchased.
2. Your rating from 1 – 5 (with 5 being the best).
3. Your feedback about the product, including how our materials helped you meet your goals and ways in which we can improve our products.
4. Your full name and shipping address so we can send your **FREE *MBLEx Essential Test Tips DVD***.

If you have any questions or concerns please feel free to contact us directly at 5star@triviumtestprep.com. Thank you, and good luck with your studies!

* Please note that the free DVD is <u>not included</u> with this book. To receive the free DVD, please follow the instructions above.

MBLEX

Terms and Definitions with
Practice Test Questions and Answers
for the Massage and Bodywork
Licensing Examination

E.M. Falgout

INTRODUCTION

Congratulations! You are one step closer to becoming a certified massage therapist. The end of examinations is in sight, and soon your practice will be in full swing.

Before you can begin your practice as a professional massage therapist, there are a few more steps to complete following massage school graduation. The MBLEx (Massage and Bodywork Licensing Examination) is one of them. After you receive confirmation that you have passed the exam, you can begin the process to become licensed to practice in your state. The licensing process varies from state to state. The best information can be found with your state's regulatory board—either online or in person, via phone or at the office.

What is a Massage Therapist?

A **massage therapist** is a professional trained in the manipulation of soft tissues of the body by stroking, rubbing, kneading, and using other techniques to encourage relaxation and healing in the client's body.

There are many different types, or modalities, of massage that massage therapists can incorporate into their practice and treatments—typically massage therapists will use a blend of their knowledge and skills to create their own treatment style. Just like other professionals, massage therapists can use their unique brand to build a client base; whether you are known for your gentle, relaxing work or your deep, therapeutic work, or perhaps a mixture of both, clients will seek you out based on your style in addition to things like your personality, work ethic, and practice space.

To become a professional massage therapist working in the United States, an individual will have to fulfill a number of requirements as described below.

QUALIFICATIONS

Requirements to become a professional massage therapist vary from state to state, and sometimes even from county to county within a state. It is very important that you know and understand the rules where you live, or where you want to practice, to ensure you have met all the requirements to practice professionally. If you have questions about requirements, you can find specific resources at your school, or you can contact the regulatory oversight body/registrar of your state.

While students entering a massage school program are encouraged to have some secondary education or some degree of professional experience, a GED or high school diploma is all that most schools require.

Most massage schools offer programs that meet, if not exceed, hours and education required by their state for licensure, in addition to providing students with the knowledge to pass the MBLEx. Hours for general massage programs can vary from 350 hours to 1,000, depending on the state. Most programs only offer the bare minimum in regards to massage education, and often certifications like prenatal and postnatal massage or hot stone massage are obtained through continuing education after a massage therapist is a practicing professional.

In addition to classroom learning, most massage schools will offer on-the-job training with externships in sports offices or spas, student clinics, and other events outside school. Students can be observed by instructors and other professionals—allowing them to get some "real world" experience while still receiving coaching from the experts. Stay organized with the following checklist:

COMMON ROLES AND RESPONSIBILITIES OF MASSAGE THERAPISTS

Being a professional massage therapist is an incredibly rewarding line of work. You get to help people who are stressed or in pain return to a more relaxed state of mind, teach them about their muscular anatomy and show them how to stretch to relieve chronically tight muscle groups, and become a constant sign of strength and peace in people's lives. It feels good!

As rewarding as the field of massage therapy can be, it also has challenges. Sometimes schedules are not right, or a person might forget his appointment; you might have a client who was not completely truthful on her intake form, or you may have a client who is inappropriate or difficult to deal with. While we always hope all clients will come fifteen minutes before their appointment, be honest with their health history, and behave kindly, we have to be prepared to deal professionally with the worst—just in case.

Excellent communication skills are of the utmost importance. You will not only appear professional, but you will also earn respect from your clients by setting boundaries. Keeping things professional can sometimes be difficult with very friendly clients who want to know more about you—where you grew up, where you live now, who you vote for, if you're seeing anyone . . . The slope can get slippery pretty quickly. Being an excellent communicator, though, you can put a stop to these comments and questions by encouraging clients to focus on their breathing, or, if that does not work, by asking them to stop or warning them you will have to stop the treatment if their prying continues.

The above is an example of being professional and keeping yourself safe. Other safety concerns may be physical; to avoid risking injury, make sure equipment is in working order and cords and other hazards are out of the way of both the client and the therapist. Communication protects clients by keeping them informed as long as you, as the therapist, describe the treatment specifically. (Please note this information is covered more in depth in chapter 3 of this review book.)

Not to be dismissed is hygiene, which is also of the utmost importance. You should maintain short, unpainted nails; keep hair out of your face; clean your body regularly; and wash your hands frequently throughout your shift, especially after each client. Also, keep in mind that what you eat emits smells from your body; if garlic chicken gives you gas, it is probably best to save that meal for after your shift is over.

The best way to deal with clients is to try to put yourself in their shoes. Yes, the client may be acting like a jerk, but on her intake form she said she has had lower back and neck pain for three months. You would probably be a little grumpy too if you were in pain that long. If all else fails, remain professional and know that after the treatment, you can suggest another therapist for her next massage.

MASSAGE THERAPY SETTINGS

A number of people still view massage as a luxury that occurs in a high-end spa. While that can be the case, there are many different settings where massage takes place.

Yes, massage can take place in a high-priced, luxury spa. Typically, these massage treatments come with flourishes, or extras, such as body wraps or facials, or hot stone treatments. Because of the setting, the experience of the therapist, and additions to the treatment, these massages are often expensive, being upward of $150 per treatment. Not only can you work in spas on land, but cruise ships also have spas—you can see the world while working.

As you are currently studying massage therapy or have just completed your training, you know that massage is much more than a relaxing treatment at a spa. Massage can also take place in a rehabilitation clinic, for clients recovering from a physical injury or an addiction. As discussed in chapter 6, compassionate touch can promote healing and serenity within the body.

Massage can also supplement chiropractic and physical therapy as part of a monthly maintenance regimen or as a temporary measure during recovering from an injury or surgery. In addition, professional and collegiate sports teams often have massage therapists on staff to ensure their players are in top-notch condition both before and after sporting events.

Sports massage, deep tissue, clinical/medical massage, oncology (cancer) massage—all of these specific, different types of massage are needed in a number of settings. Massage therapy is a growing field with a wide range of opportunity and advancement in a number of different areas.

In addition to the physical practice of performing massage, there are plenty of other jobs within massage, from teaching general massage courses or continuing education classes to writing about massage for magazines or even test preparation books like this one. The world of massage is rich with possibilities!

THE FUTURE OF MASSAGE THERAPY

The world of massage is far reaching and ever expanding. As the field gains more credibility with national certification standards like the MBLEx and state licensing, opportunities for therapists grow. Some insurance carriers even cover massage therapy in clinical settings; due to the affordability of such coverage, more people are being drawn to massage as clients. Additionally, many clients are looking for a holistic health approach, using massage along with a healthy diet and exercise to maintain a balanced lifestyle.

Furthermore, medical professionals are increasingly looking to massage therapists to help their patients with pain management or in palliative care, though there are some out there who still view massage as a luxury.

While it is great news for you as a therapist that the world of massage therapy is growing and advancing, it also means that with the change and growth will come new challenges. Therapists are responsible for individual professional development. More reputable institutions are turning out massage therapists ready to grow and advance the industry. Massage therapists must uphold a high level of professionalism to maintain and increase the respect and validity paid to the field and their work.

National Certification

Massage, like any other trade profession, needs to have rules, regulations, and standards of education that can be measured to ensure that individual professionalism is maintained. The MBLEx is the national certification that measures these standards in the world of massage.

WHAT IS THE MBLEx?

The MBLEx is maintained and administered by the Federation of State Massage Therapy Boards (FSMTB). The FSMTB's mission is to support member boards in the work so that the practice of massage therapy is provided to the public in a safe and effective manner. The FSMTB developed the MBLEx to "offer the first standardized licensing exam for the massage and bodywork profession; to facilitate professional mobility; to give the regulatory community oversight over exam content, organizational policies and procedures pertaining to the exam; and to significantly speed up the process between application and examination to avoid unnecessary delays in licensure."

Think of it like this: passing the MBLEx and getting licensed establishes your credibility as a massage therapist in your community. Your clients will see your credentials and be confident that you know what you are doing in providing their treatment.

There are two different ways to sign up to take the MBLEx: through the FSMTB or through your state's licensing board or agency. To go through the FSMTB, sign up for the exam at the official website: https://www.fsmtb.org/mblex/application-process/. After you verify that you have completed all the necessary education, agree to the test's policies in writing, and pay the fee of $195, you'll receive an "Authorization to Test" (ATT) via email. You must sign up to take the test within ninety days at Pearson Vue: http://www.pearsonvue.com/fsmtb/. If you need to change locations or your testing date, you can contact Pearson Vue as well.

Should you go through your state's licensing board or agency, you must first be approved by that organization; the same steps as above apply in terms of signing off on the test, paying the fee, and scheduling the exam.

Each multiple-choice question is worth one raw point. The total number of questions you answer correctly is added up to obtain your raw score, which is then converted to a number on a scale of 300 – 900. In order to pass the MBLEx, you must receive at least a score of 630.

The score will be kept electronically, but you can request a physical copy for a $20 fee.

Either route you take will allow you to move toward being a licensed professional therapist after you pass—it really just depends on how your school or state does things. One option is no better than the other; what you choose may be based on preference and availability of services in your area.

WHAT YOU NEED TO LEARN TO PASS THE MBLEX

The breakdown of the exam follows in the table below. While it may seem like an overwhelming amount of information, there are only 100 questions to be answered in two hours. Think back to your days in massage school, and use this test prep as a road map for your success.

Everything from muscle actions, origins, and insertions to asking your clients about their health history will be on the exam. Remember to breathe.

CONTINUE

What's on the MBLEx?

Topic	Content	Percent of Test	Number of Questions*
Body Systems	Anatomy and Physiology	12%	11 – 13
	Kinesiology	11%	10 – 12
Pathology	Pathology, Contra-indications, Special Populations, Areas of Caution	13%	12 – 15
Application	Benefits and Physiological Effects of Techniques That Manipulate Soft Tissue	14%	13 – 16
Assessment	Client Assessment, Reassessment, and Treatment Planning	17%	16 – 18
CAM (Complimentary and Alternative Medicines)	Overview of Massage and Bodywork Modalities/Culture/History	5%	4 – 6
Professional	Ethics, Boundaries, Laws, Regulations	15%	14 – 17
	Guidelines for Professional Practice	13%	12 – 15

*numbers are approximate

WHAT TO EXPECT ON TESTING DAY

You do not have to dread test day anymore! You have put hours, days, weeks, and months into preparing for this exam, and this book is designed to make sure you know your stuff—which you do!

Now that you know you have the material down, here is what you need to know for the logistical side of taking this exam:

- Arrive at least thirty minutes early in the event there is a delay, and to ensure you are not feeling rushed before the start of the exam.

- Bring only what you need. Most things, such as a watch, phone, chewing gum, etc., will not be allowed into the exam room. Lockers will be provided for keys or jackets.

- Two forms of valid identification are required. Check https://www.fsmtb.org/ to be sure you have the most up-to-date information.

You will not be able to flag questions for review at a later time. If you need to use the bathroom, you may raise your hand, but it is better to go before the exam begins as the time does not stop for your breaks.

Since the test is computerized, it will base your questions on how well you are doing in the exam. If you answer a question correctly, then the next question will be of the same or higher difficulty level, but if you answer a question incorrectly, the following question will be easier. This pattern continues throughout the test.

After answering 100 questions in (under) two hours, you can notify the official that you are finished with the exam, and your score will be waiting for you at the front where you checked in.

AFTER YOU PASS THE MBLEX

You did it! You are now a CMT, or certified massage therapist. Now you have to register with your state licensing board so you can practice professionally. Most states require licenses to be renewed every two years, for a fee, in addition to a certain number of continuing education (CE) hours. As always, it is important to check with your state licensing board to make sure you have everything necessary for the initial license and then for the following renewal years.

Continuing education courses allow you to build your skill set and open your practice to a new level of clientele. Also, it is good for professionals to constantly be learning and practicing their skills on other professionals to get productive feedback.

The world of professional massage therapy is now open to you! Go forth and prosper!

Effleurage

Friction

Petrissage

a gliding, stroking, and light touch technique

a technique used to break up existing and forming adhesions in muscles, tendons, and ligaments

a kneading technique

Tapotement

Vibration

Code of Ethics

a technique also referred to as *percussion*

a technique that is rapid and rhythmical while maintaining constant contact

establishes professional conduct, behavior, and acceptable application of services provided by a professional

Self-Accountability

Competence

Informed Consent

behaving with integrity in the absence of external authority

honestly practicing skills learned from school and continuing education

type of consent that MUST be obtained before a massage can proceed

Dual Relationship

What is the Health Insurance Portability and Accountability Act (HIPAA)?

SOAP Notes

when a therapist-client relationship overlaps with a relationship outside of the therapeutic session

a national standard of practices for the electronic exchange, privacy, and security of health information

a chart primarily used in outcome-based massage

Hydrocollator

What is the purpose of the Occupational Safety and Health Administration (OSHA)?

Erythrocytes

a gel-filled pack in a metal tank filled with temperature-controlled water

Its mission is to "save lives, prevent injuries, and protect the health of America's workers."

red blood cells

Eukocytes

Thrombocytes (Platelets)

Aorta

white blood cells

fragmented cells that prevent hemorrhaging

the primary artery that starts the systemic circuit

Superior Vena Cava

Inferior Vena Cava

What are the three layers of artery and vein walls?

collects blood from the head, neck, chest, and upper extremities

collects blood from the pelvic and abdominal region and lower extremities

tunica intima, tunica media, and tunica externa

Vasodilation

Vasoconstriction

Capillary Exchange

enlargement of diameter of artery and vein walls

narrowing of diameter of artery and vein walls

a process that delivers nutrients and oxygen while picking up cell waste

Purkinje Fibers

Hyperemia

Ischemia

fibers that cause impulses to spread throughout the ventricular myocardium

when skin becomes red and warm as a result of increased blood flow

caused when blood flow to an organ is inadequate or interrupted

What are the most common blood types?

Universal Donors

Universal Recipients

A, B, O

those with type-O blood; their blood can be used by recipients of any blood type

those with type-AB blood; they can receive any type of blood

Alimentary Canal

Gastrointestinal (GI) Tract

Bolus

a canal in the digestive system that begins with ingestion and ends at excretion

another name for the alimentary canal

a masticated lump formed during digestion

Chyme

Villi

Ileum

a semifluid mass passed to the small intestine

small fingerlike projections that line the small intestine

a section of the small intestine that contains clusters of lacteals that enhance fat absorption

Colon

Accessory Organs

Bile

Its primary purpose is to transport, store, and excrete indigestible material.

salivary glands, liver, gallbladder, and pancreas

produced by the liver, an emulsifier that breaks apart large fat globules

Hormones

What are the three mechanisms that control the level of hormones secreted into the bloodstream?

Pineal Gland

chemical messengers

Negative Feedback, Hormonal Control, Neural Control

a pinecone-shaped gland located behind the brain's thalamus that produces melatonin and regulates the pituitary gland

Keratin

Melanin

Collagen

a protein that waterproofs and protects the skin

provides UV protection and determines skin pigment

a group of structural proteins found in skin, ligaments, blood vessels, and bones

Sudoriferous Glands

Sebum

Hair Follicles

glands that excrete sweat

an oily substance that lubricates and waterproofs the skin and hair

small tube-shaped craters contained in the epidermis

Arrector Pili

Nail Matrix

Eponychium

small muscles that hold hair follicles in place

a vascular layer of cells that nourish the nail root

commonly known as the cuticle

What are the four phases of skin healing?

Angiogenesis

Primary Lymphatic Structures

inflammatory, epithelialization, proliferative, remodeling

the formation of new blood vessels

bone marrow and thymus

Spleen

Peyer's Patches

What collects lymph draining from the abdomen and lower body?

the largest lymphatic organ

nodules found in the mucous membrane of the small intestine

Cisterna Chyli

Sarcomeres

What protein resembles a twisted double strand of beads and aids in muscle contraction?

What protein appears as small heads with elongated tails and aids in muscle contraction?

bundles of myofibrils in parallel rows

Actin

Myosin

What are the two types of protein molecules that cover actin?

Neuromuscular Junction

This energy-carrying molecule is formed when adenosine diphosphate (ADP) and phosphate molecules become energized.

Troponin and Tropomyosin

where the synapse and muscle fibers meet

Adenosine Triphosphate (ATP)

Central Nervous System

Peripheral Nervous System

Which system controls voluntary and involuntary skeletal muscle contractions?

the nervous system that contains the brain and spinal cord

the nervous system that contains cranial and spinal nerves

Somatic Nervous System

Which system controls subconscious glandular secretions and contraction of cardiac and smooth muscle?

Sympathetic Nervous System

Parasympathetic Nervous System

Autonomic Nervous System

the *fight-or-flight* nervous system

the *rest-and-digest* nervous system

Neurons

Neuroglia

What term refers to signals that travel down axons?

cells that send and receive stimuli

cells that support and protect neurons

Nerve Impulse Conduction

Afferent Nerves

Efferent Nerves

What are the two ions that go into action during nerve transmission and muscle contraction?

nerves that receive sensory information to send to the brain

nerves that receive motor signals from the brain

Sodium and Potassium

What are the six types of neuroglia?

What are the four regions of the brain?

Saltatory Signals

Astrocytes, Ependymal, Microglia, Oligodendrocytes, Satellite, Schwann

Cerebrum, Cerebellum, Diencephalon, Brain Stem

signals conducted down myelinated axons

Continuous Signals

Nodes of Ranvier

Cerebrum

signals conducted down unmyelinated axons

the gaps along myelinated axons

the largest region of the brain

Corpus Callosum

Occipital Lobe

Diencephalon

a communication pathway between the two hemispheres of the brain

the brain lobe involved in reading and writing comprehension

the brain region that houses the thalamus and hypothalamus

Brain Stem

Reflex Arc

Autonomic Reflex

the brain region that consists of the midbrain and hindbrain

a neural pathway that allows the body to respond without delay

the reflex that maintains homeostasis (such as the heart beating)

Olfactory Nerve

Optic Nerve

Trachea

the cranial nerve related to smell

the cranial nerve related to vision

commonly referred to as the windpipe

Hyaline Cartilage

Alveolar Sacs

What term describes the greatest volume of air that can be pulled into an individual's lungs?

c-shaped rings in the trachea

sacs located at the end of each bronchiole

vital capacity

What are the five types of connective bone tissue?

Where is bone marrow found?

What are the five classifications of bones?

Osseous, Cartilage, Ligaments, Periosteum, Bone Marrow

Medullary Cavity of Long Bones

Long, Short, Flat, Sesamoid, Irregular

Diaphysis

Short Bone

Flat Bone

the name of a long bone shaft

the bone classification of carpals and tarsals

the bone classification of the scapula

Patella

Axial and Appendicular

In the bone remodeling process, these form new bone.

the largest sesamoid bone in the human body

the two skeletal regions of the human body

osteoblasts

In the bone remodeling process, these break down bone.

What are mature bone cells called?

What is the condition that may result when bone breaks down faster than it is rebuilt?

osteoclasts

osteocytes

osteoporosis

What are distinguishing features of bones called?

What are the three classifications of joints?

What is another word for *joint*?

bony landmarks

synarthrotic, amphiarthrotic, diarthrotic

articulation

What is an alternative name for a diarthrotic joint?

What are the three classifications of diarthrotic joints?

Bursae

synovial joint

monoaxial, biaxial, triaxial

fluid-filled pockets related to articulations

What are the two types of immune responses?

What are the two types of cells involved in the adaptive immune response?

Kidneys

innate and adaptive response

t lymphocytes (t-cells) and b lymphocytes (b-cells)

a pair of bean-shaped organs that filter waste and excess fluid from blood to produce urine

Ureters

Urethra

Qi

tubes that extend from each kidney

receives the urine from the urinary bladder

energy of the universe or life energy

Each of these peak for a two-hour period during a cycle.

What is the concept behind yin and yang?

Ayurvedic System

meridian channels

the belief that the mind, body, spirit, and the entire universe are interconnected and inseparable

a health and treatment system derived from and developed in India's Vedic culture

What are the three doshas in the Ayurvedic system?

These relate to areas that run along the midline and are associated with organs, systems, and anatomical locations.

In English, this means *finger pressure*.

Vata, Pitta, Kapha

chakras

shiatsu

These therapies have roots in Eastern medicine, holistic nursing, and osteopathy.

What are the twelve channels in traditional Chinese medicine?

This meridian channel's primary function is to circulate source qi to all organs.

light touch/energy healing

meridians

triple warmer

Bladder Meridian Channel

This meridian channel is considered the root of life and stores essence.

What are the five elements in Ayurveda?

the longest meridian channel

kidney meridian channel

air, ether, fire, water, and earth

What are the five elements in traditional Chinese medicine?

What are the assessment tools in traditional Chinese medicine?

This word means *dark side of the mountain.*

metal, earth, fire, water, and wood

looking, listening, smelling, asking, and palpation

yin

This word means *sun side of the mountain.*

Kinesiology

These muscles appear feathery and have a central tendon.

yang

the scientific study of the movement of the human body

pennate muscles

Sphincters are classified as what type of muscle?

The rectus abdominis is classified as what type of muscle?

Convergent Muscles

circular muscles

parallel muscles

muscles that are triangular in shape

Proprioceptors

Muscle Spindles

Golgi Tendon Organs

sensory receptors that communicate speed, angles, and balance to the central nervous system

proprioceptors that sense muscle stretching

proprioceptors that sense muscle tension

How is range of motion (ROM) defined in kinesiology?

What are the four muscles of the rotator cuff?

What are the three columns of muscles in the erector spinae group?

active, passive, and resistive

teres minor, infraspinatus, supraspinatus, subscapularis

iliocostalis, longissimus, spinalis

What muscles assist only with inhalation and exhalation?

What are the five muscles involved in moving the mandible?

What are the four key muscles for neck flexion, rotation, and elevation of the ribs?

external and internal intercostals; serratus posterior, superior, and inferior

masseter, temporalis, lateral and medial pterygoid, platysma

anterior, middle, and posterior scalene, and the sternocleido-mastoid (SCM)

What are the two types of muscular contractions in kinesiology?

Muscle Cramp

Muscle Spasm

isometric and isotonic

an involuntary contraction of the muscle

an involuntary contraction neurological in nature

What are the three phases of skeletal muscle injury healing?

A primary tenet of this treatment is to improve communication between the muscles and the nervous system.

What are the two types of proprioceptive neuromuscular facilitation (PNF) stretches?

inflammatory, repair, and remodeling

proprioceptive neuromuscular facilitation (PNF)

PNF hold-relax, PNF contract-relax

What is the term in kinesiology for a type of skeletal muscle fibers found in red meat?

What is the term in kinesiology for a combination of red and white skeletal muscle fibers?

What is the term in kinesiology for fibers that are white in appearance?

slow twitch fibers

fast twitch A fibers

fast twitch B fibers

Pacinian Corpuscles

Levers

What are the three main roles of muscles when joint movement occurs?

corpuscles that respond to quick and fleeting touch and vibration

The skeletal and muscular system work together to produce joint movement using this concept.

prime mover, synergist, antagonist

What are the three aspects of a lever?

Passive Range of Motion

Resistive Range of Motion

load, fulcrum, force

when a therapist can move a joint without assistance from the client

when a force is applied to create resistance, resulting in increased strength, flexibility, and improved range of motion

Aneurysm

Arteriosclerosis

Atherosclerosis

considered a silent killer, an outward bulge in a vessel or heart

hardening of the arteries and reduction in arterial elasticity

a buildup of plaque in the arteries and thickening of the arterial wall

Asthma

Chronic Obstructive Pulmonary Disease
(COPD)

Deep Vein Thrombosis (DVT)

when smooth muscle of the bronchial tubes spasms and con-
stricts in response to an allergen, stress, or inflammation

a collection of chronic lung conditions

an inflammation of a deep vein caused by a blood clot

Diabetes Mellitus

Embolism

This disease may occur when stomach acids backsplash into the esophagus.

a chronic inability of the body to produce insulin to properly metabolize carbohydrates; classified as type 1 and type 2

a blood clot or gas bubble that moves throughout the circulatory system

Gastroesophageal Reflux Disease (GERD)

Hyperthyroidism

This autoimmune condition occurs when the synovial fluid in a joint is attacked by the immune system.

Transient Ischemic Attack (TIA)

an overproduction of thyroid-producing hormones

Rheumatoid Arthritis (RA)

when a small blood clot blocks the flow of blood to the brain for a brief period

Whiplash

What disorder is commonly referred to as *frozen shoulder*?

What syndrome is caused by compression of the median nerve by the transverse carpal ligament?

when tendons, muscles, and ligaments in and around the neck are sprained or strained by a violent thrusting

Adhesive Capsulitis

Carpal Tunnel Syndrome

What is the term for a pressure ulcer or bedsore?

Edema

This disease results from an excess amount of uric acid and is clinically referred to as *hyperuricemia*.

Decubitus Ulcer

the accumulation of interstitial fluid in the lymphatic and circu-latory capillaries

Gout

Hernia

This virus can cause blisters around the mouth, lips, genitals, thighs, and buttocks.

This disease is also known as *wear-and-tear* arthritis.

a protrusion of an organ through the membrane that encases it

herpes simplex

osteoarthritis

Shin Splints

Sciatic Nerve

Squamous Cell Carcinoma

pain resulting from microscopic tears and inflammation of the fascia and periosteum of the tibia

the nerve that runs under or through the piriformis muscle

presents as a scaly red patch, an open sore, and elevated growth that crusts and bleeds

Scoliosis

Tinea

Varicose Vein

a curvature of the spine most frequently to the right and most common in females

a lesion caused by a fungal infection and may be referred to as ringworm, jock itch, or athlete's foot

a superficial vein that becomes twisted and swollen because of damaged or weakened vessel valves

Homeostasis

What massage modality combines massage, stretching, energy flow, and a genuine client-centered intent?

Trigger Points

the ability of the body to regulate equilibrium or balance across all systems

Thai massage

hyperirritable spots, or knots, in taut bands of muscle

In which massage modality do therapists use their feet?

Which massage modality originated in Hawaiian and Polynesian cultures?

Which massage modality uses therapeutic-grade essential oils applied in a sequence along the spine?

Ashiatsu

Lomi Lomi

Raindrop Therapy

Watsu®

Thermotherapy

What are the three ways heat can travel from one source to another?

a water-based treatment that incorporates shiatsu techniques

the transfer of heat in hydrotherapy

conduction, convection, and radiation

What term describes cold therapy?

Blood-Borne Pathogens

cryotherapy

infectious microorganisms in human blood that can cause disease in humans

Made in the USA
Coppell, TX
07 April 2022

76170963R00083